The Litter Patrol Workout

staying fit while doing good

Fírinn Taisdeal

Dedication

To all the litterbugs who helped me stay in tip-top shape.

Table of Contents

1. How the Litter Patrol Workout came about

Litter is everywhere. It's on our streets, our beaches, in city parks, strewn all over vacant lots. You will find litter on remote trails, along the edge of secluded lakes, blowing all over the desert, at the tops of glorious mountains, and in the corners of nearly every parking lot. There is litter all over the ocean, all over the world. Litter of the ugliest kind clogs lovely stream beds, and turns otherwise beautiful scenic overlooks into a spectacle of discarded plastic bags, beer cans, styrofoam cups, cigarette cartons, cigarette butts, whiskey bottles, and worse. Almost anywhere you go, you will find litter of all different kinds, making everyone's experience of our world a little bit more depressing, certainly uglier, and raising serious questions about the species of which we are all members, *homo sapiens*, the species which should know better.

I have a detailed knowledge of litter, because I've been picking it up my entire life, all over the world. I do this for one fundamental reason: because it makes life a little better for all of us. When I was a boy, my father planted an idea in my mind which he expressed in simple terms in our household:

When you leave a room, you should have made the room a little bit better than when you entered.

As this idea percolated within my young mind, I began applying it in other ways. I began thinking of every place I went as a "room," which I could try to make a little bit better. Whenever I took a walk, each new location was a new "room" I was entering. I was thankful for all the interesting and wonderful places I walked, and I wanted to express my love for those places–and litter was everywhere I went. The way to improve those places could not have been more obvious. So I began picking up litter wherever I walked. It was never a burden to do so. I was happy to express my thanks to every location I enjoyed, and even to some I didn't enjoy, but that someone should clean up anyway.

I began to do this regularly. I invented all kinds of techniques and tricks to make the process effective and efficient. I learned to deal with all kinds of litter, and all different environments. Eventually, I had done this so many times, in so many locations and in so many ways, that I became an expert, with knowledge both broad and deep of the peculiarly ubiquitous phenomenon of litter.

1

I also began to notice that this activity was excellent exercise. If I started to clean up a site, within only a few minutes I had a good sweat going, and my heart rate was elevated. Because I exercise regularly in other ways, I knew from experience that cleaning up litter could be very good exercise. I began to wonder why I was paying for a gym membership and driving to the gym, only to exert myself on some artificial machines, doing absolutely no good for anyone else–not even generating electricity from my exertions, just moving a part of a machine back and forth rather senselessly, and not even out in the fresh air. While on my litter patrols I would see people running by, getting exercise, but I was getting exercise and doing good at the same time, while they were just running. I also began to notice that the exercise I was getting picking up litter was actually better than running, because I was using many different muscles, the activity was tremendously varied, and I often had to exercise my balance in reaching for items. I then began to experiment with truly demanding forms of the Litter Patrol Workout, combining picking up litter with running, stretching, and bodyweight exercises. Using the Litter Patrol Workout I had devised, I got into amazing shape, the best shape of my life. I began to imagine a world in which so many people began picking up litter while exercising that litter became rare, instead of ubiquitous, and everyone who did so was also in better shape.

Sure, that ideal sounds a bit nutty, but it actually could happen, and it would be wonderful. I invite you to become part of a positive change in society, a change which would be good in every way, and a change of which you could be proud, if you choose to participate.

2. Who the heck litters?

I have a confession to make. I'm still completely puzzled as to who litters, and why they do it. It seems crazy to me that anyone would just toss a piece of trash where it will clearly be an eyesore for everyone else, possibly for years to come. Littering seems even more crazy to me when I witness just how close litter baskets often are to large collections of litter. What that means is that people who litter aren't even willing to take a few seconds to walk over to a nearby litter basket. To me, that is just plain weird and despicable

I find the ubiquity of litter even more puzzling when I consider how infrequently I ever witness someone littering. Litter is everywhere, but you almost never see someone in the act of littering. It is therefore reasonable to conclude that not that many people are litterbugs. The proportion of the population that litters is very small, but accounts for nearly all of the litter. It's highly likely that this small proportion of the population is completely incorrigible. They have always littered, and they always will. My own conclusion is that littering will always be with us, and that anti-littering campaigns are probably a complete waste of time and resources. It would be nice to think otherwise, but we've had millennia to solve the problem of littering, and it's no closer to being solved than it was fifty, a hundred or a thousand years ago.

Does that mean that the litterbugs are solely responsible for the ubiquity of litter? My own surprising answer to that question is in the next section.

3. Who the heck doesn't pick it up?

Since the litterbugs will never stop being litterbugs, but the proportion of the population that are litterbugs is very small, the reason there is still litter everywhere is very simple:

Because everyone else never bothers to pick it up.

The number of people who don't litter is much greater than the people who do litter, but the proportion of people who never pick litter up is close to 100%. People who don't litter outnumber people who do litter by a factor of at least ten to one, so the non-litterers could make all the litter disappear with only a minor effort. In addition, litterbugs are leaving litter at a rate that is much slower than that of someone who deliberately picks litter up; a litterbug might leave a few items a day, but in half an hour one person could easily pick up dozens and dozens of pieces of litter. Put all this together, and it is completely clear that the continuing presence of litter everywhere is actually the fault of the people who don't bother to pick it up.

My ultimate goal is to not only convince you to begin picking up litter regularly, and get some great exercise while doing so, but to convince you to also convince other people to do the same. Together, we can make a small but significant improvement to society, and make nearly everywhere we travel look a little bit better.

4. Show your love by removing litter

I know many people who love nature, and hate litter, but also never bother to clean any of it up. This causes me to question just how deep their love of nature really is, and perhaps to conclude that their "love" of nature extends only to enjoying nature, using nature, taking from nature, but never giving back, never caring enough to make an effort. True love means being willing to make an effort. The same idea applies to any location you care about, and applies to society, and to humanity.

If you care about your city, show your love by cleaning it up. If you care about your suburban neighborhood, show your love by cleaning it up. If you care about other people, show your love by making more enjoyable and more beautiful the places they spend time. If you care about humanity, care enough to maintain an inspiring environment, and be a good example in every way you can.

5. Join a special group of people

At the moment, there are very few people living the "litter picker upper" way of life, and even fewer people adding excellent exercise into the mix. Those few of us who pick up litter because we believe it's the right thing to do are a very special group of people. I've been picking up litter actively for years, and I have only met a few other people who also do this, but those people were truly exceptional as people: exceptionally nice, exceptionally ethical, exceptionally open and exceptionally positive in their outlook. It's always fun meeting others who have had the same realizations you have had, in this case the realization that there is a simple way to make the world a little better for everyone, and get some fresh air and exercise while you're at it.

If you begin going out on litter patrol, you may never encounter another person doing what you are doing. You may get people saying "thank you" as they pass by, people honking and waving in appreciation, but chances are you won't encounter another dedicated litter picker up, let alone one who gets regular, fine exercise this way. Don't worry about it. The truth is that there *are* other people to do this (the author is obviously one), and you are part of a special group of responsible, caring citizens doing good in a direct way in the world, and possibly inspiring others. If you can recruit your friends and make a fun social activity of it, all the better.

6. Litter Patrol as a way of life

Joining the Litter Patrol team is actually a way of life, a way of seeing the world, and an enhanced way of relating to your physical environment. Litter Patrol is also moral outlook, a way of taking on a specific, ongoing responsibility, as well as a way of deepening the way you relate to society, to nature, and to the qualities of courage and creativity. At this point, you may of course be wondering what courage and creativity have to do with just picking up some trash, so let me explain in full.

If you begin going out on Litter Patrol, you are definitely doing something unusual, something that very few people do. You may feel like you're being a weirdo. You may feel like you're doing something "uncool." That's part of precisely what's wonderful about it. You're actually being a rebel. You're going against the usual patterns, and you're definitely going to stand out. To go out on Litter Patrol, and do it proudly, you have to have some social courage, or develop some. But you know you're making the world a little bit better, you know you're being a good example, and you know if more people did this that it would be wonderful, and people would have more confidence in each other, and in society. That's a lot to be proud of. So be courageous, go out and be obviously different, and do so proudly.

Litter Patrol is also inherently creative, in a couple of ways. First, if you're not at all used to the idea of going out picking up litter, it's an act of creativity in itself to engage in a new activity, and explore its various aspects. Litter Patrol is also creative in that you will find yourself noticing areas which could use some attention, you will learn surprising things about those areas when you engage with them, and you may also learn some surprising things about yourself. Those new experiences will enhance your creativity. In addition, you will inevitably develop your own way of going about Litter Patrol, and doing so involves being creative.

7. Don't by shy, and don't be proud in the wrong way

Some people have the odd idea that it is beneath them to pick up litter. They think doing so is the sole responsibility of civic authorities, or they may have an even worse attitude. "Garbage is for the garbage men," they say. "That's why we pay our taxes," they say. That's precisely the attitude that makes litter so prevalent, and makes many different environments unpleasant to look at and discouraging to think about. Behind that attitude is often a belief that picking up litter is somehow an inherently undignified activity, reserved only for a lower class, the "garbage men."

I think the opposite is true. I think stepping forward and taking responsibility for solving a problem is inherently dignified, inherently worthy, and to be admired. If you have any notion that picking up litter is somehow embarrassing or beneath you, I would encourage you to reverse your views, and take pride in doing something helpful, and take pride in being one of the few people with the insight to take on the task. Don't be shy. Be proud of making a great choice, from which everyone benefits.

8. Adventures in litter patrol around the world

As I said, I've been doing Litter Patrol for many years now, ever since I was a teenager. I grew up in a town in Connecticut which was relatively clean, and had many beautiful natural sites, but I would often find lots of litter in even the nicest natural sites, so I would clean those sites up. I walked many a mile in that town, picking up litter wherever I went.

When I moved to the San Francisco Bay Area, I continued my activities. I used to live on a gritty street in San Francisco, and about once a week I would clean up the entire street, to the amazement of the neighborhood. I took up sea kayaking in San Francisco Bay, and got extra exercise pursuing floating debris and hauling it into the kayak or lashing it to the deck, then disposing of it properly on land. On backpacking trips, I would bring an extra couple of plastic bags, and pick up anything that didn't belong out in such beautiful, natural settings.

Next I began doing Litter Patrol while traveling in the U.S. One day while on Litter Patrol in Stockbridge, Massachusetts I noticed that a certain area was unusually clean. Soon I discovered the reason: another member of the worldwide Litter Patrol team! She lives in town, and told me that she cleans up the area completely every day, down to the last cigarette butt. We had a great conversation, and it was wonderful to meet another member of the team.

On vacation, I had some reluctance at first to engage in Litter Patrol, particularly in foreign countries where I didn't know how it would be taken culturally. I started in Puerto Rico. Let me tell you, that place is a big, litter-infested mess. I don't know what those people think they're doing down there, but in so many parts of Puerto Rico they are turning a beautiful island into a garbage dump. I did the best I could, cleaning up beaches, and even city streets. I went about this proudly, even amid stares and laughter. It was great.

The Litter Patrol Workout

On vacation, I make sure I have a good time, but I also make sure I go out on Litter Patrol wherever I am, no matter what the natives think. One day while waiting for a train in Trieste, Italy, I realized I had time to clean up nearly the entire area outside the train station. So that's what I did, with a bunch of Italians and Slovenians clearly wondering if I was a madman. I just smiled, and went about my business, and about an hour later the Trieste train station was cleaner than it had been in years.

On the island of Mali Losinj in Croatia at the end of the summer all the tourists had left, leaving all their litter behind. Mali Losinj is a beautiful place, set in the deep blue of the Adriatic Sea. It also the home of my Croat ancestors, and so has a special meaning for me. It was upsetting to see such a beautiful place ruined by litter, so of course I set to work, and I'm glad I did. In the process of hunting down pieces of litter in various crevices on the rocky beaches, I encountered all kinds of wonderful, minute aspects of nature I otherwise would never have noticed, never seen up close. I met tiny lizards face to face, got to know the local seaweed in intimate detail, and studied the lichenous deposits on the rocks–all while under observation by the many local feral cats. I cleaned up a beautiful cove, all the details of which I will remember happily for the rest of my life.

One of the funniest experiences was in Russia. I had been traveling by bus from Moscow to a small village about eight hours out in the countryside. We stopped at a large rest stop for lunch, and I soon set about Litter Patrol. The site was horrendous. I had gloves on, but I picked up some pretty gruesome stuff. The Russians are particularly egregious in their litter, I must say. After only a few minutes nearly everyone from the bus was watching me, because clearly they had never seen anything like this before, in all of Russia. Eventually one of the people walked toward me, and said, in Russian, "May I ask you a question?" I looked up, smiling, and said "Of course."

"Do you know how big this country is?"

At that point, everybody started laughing uproariously, all in good humor, and it was time to get back on the bus. It was an absolutely great experience.

Litter Patrol while traveling is a great choice to make. You will get to know the area in a way completely unlike the typical, shallow tourism, and you will find your experience deepened immensely. If you are American, and this is known as you go out on Litter Patrol in foreign lands, you may also give them a very different impression of Americans, in a most wonderful way.

9. Introduction to the Litter Patrol Workout

The essential message bears repeating; the Litter Patrol Workout is a great way to get exercise while doing good. You may care more about doing good, or you may care more about exercise, but the Litter Patrol Workout will always give you both. There are many ways of going about litter patrol, and many ways of getting a workout, so when you combine them you get even more possibilities. However, unlike certain other workout routines, the Litter Patrol Workout is always a general workout. You will not be getting bulging biceps, nor will you automatically be able to run a half marathon just from the Litter Patrol Workout. If you do the workout even in its most basic form though, you will be getting good exercise which includes some cardio, a bit of stretching in the form of reaching. You will be using many different muscle groups because of the range of movement involved, as well as exercising your balance, again because of the range of movement involved. Even the lightest form of the workout will elevate your heart rate and breathing, and cause you to sweat a bit. The more advanced forms of the workout are truly strenuous, and will put you in amazing shape.

The nature and frequency of your workouts is up to you, and partly depend on what your immediate neighborhood is like, how much you're willing to travel to specific sites, and what sorts of sites you're willing to take on. Litter patrol can be a matter of a regular schedule, or a matter of opportunity, whim and inspiration, or careful planning for major projects. Obviously, you can also combine Litter Patrol Workouts with other exercise routines for variety and cross-training, as well as incorporate other exercises within the workout. Options for getting a more challenging workout are described below under the heading "Levels & forms of the Litter Patrol Workout." What the Litter Patrol Workout will always give you is a chance to feel good about doing some good, get some exercise, be outdoors, explore new areas, get some sun, make some discoveries, and possibly inspire others.

If you go out for a walk you're already used to, but add litter patrol to that walk, you will quickly notice that the extra effort of bending down and reaching involves completely different muscles than just walking. You will definitely notice the extra exertion over the course of your walk. Where perhaps before you didn't sweat during that walk, you may begin to sweat. Your awareness of litter will increase radically. You will also notice that some litter is obvious and easy to reach, and other litter is not so easy to reach, and retrieving that litter may take you off the common paths a bit, or even a lot. You will have to make decisions about what litter you're going to go after, and what you're going to leave alone.

Another aspect of awareness you will discover is that going after pieces of litter often brings you to locations and perspectives you would otherwise never experience; if you normally just walk along a path, not noticing very much, once you spot a piece of litter you may have to go off the path, scramble a bit, reach, and all of a sudden you're looking at everything along that spot in the path in a new way, and seeing things you never saw before. It's important to learn to enjoy this fundamental aspect of the Litter Patrol Workout. If you clean up the same spot multiple times, you will develop an intimate knowledge of all the details of that spot, from all different perspectives. This is something to be savored, and cherished. It also contains lessons to keep in mind for all of life:

- You may think you know an area, but there is always so much more to know and experience about it.
- Even a slight change of perspective changes your experience, and the way you think about a place.
- Your habits and patterns, if never disrupted, can prevent you from increasing your understanding and appreciation, of places, people, and more.

10. Approaches to the Litter Patrol Workout

How you approach the Litter Patrol Workout is entirely your choice, but I'd like to describe some options that may not have occurred to you.

One approach, the simplest of all and probably the best for beginning to experiment with the Litter Patrol Workout, is to use a walking route you already know, but add litter patrol to your walk. In this case, all you do is bring a couple of bags with you when you head out on that walk, keep an eye out for litter, grab it, and bag it. If this is a regular walking route for you already, you can take satisfaction in having made the route a little nicer for yourself and others.

An entirely different approach to the Litter Patrol Workout is to keep an eye out for an area that could use a good, thorough cleanup, and then schedule a time to take care of it. If you choose to do this, you can then decide whether your goal will be to clean up the area completely, or only spend a certain amount of time on it. It's easy to underestimate how long it will take to clean up an area. Either approach is fine. Just decide which works best for you.

If you are a runner or jogger, though it might sound strange, you can actually incorporate litter patrol into your regular jogging or running routine, and you will actually get a fundamentally better, more thorough workout by doing so. Your regular route will suddenly become more demanding because of the use of different sets of muscles, and using your muscles in different ways. Combining running or jogging with litter patrol gives you exercise more akin to soccer or rugby, but even better because of the aspect of bending and reaching. Even if you are skeptical of this or it sounds funny to you, I'd suggest you give it a try, at least a couple of times. You will probably be amazed by the enhanced workout you get.

Yet another approach to the Litter Patrol workout is to be ready for a workout whenever you are on a road trip. Just keep some bags, gloves and appropriate clothes in your car, and when you find a spot and are ready for a workout, go for it. I've done this a whole lot. My favorite method is to locate an otherwise beautiful roadside pullout that has been trashed, and make it pristine again. I once did this in Western Massachusetts by an absolutely beautiful stream, spending about an hour on the site and getting gloriously sweaty, while getting to know the site in intimate detail. I actually pulled so much litter out of that site that it filled two entire trash bags. I drove on further to a small restaurant with a dumpster out back, told them what I had done, and they were happy to let me toss everything in the dumpster because they knew that particular roadside pullout, and were glad someone had cleaned it up.

11. Levels & forms of the Litter Patrol Workout

The Litter Patrol Workout can be anything from a slightly enhanced form of taking an easy walk to something approaching Iron Man training. What you make of it is up to you, but I'd like to present some options.

It's an easy matter to just stroll along, picking up any litter you encounter. This is only slightly more demanding than just walking. If you turn your walking into "power walking," and pick up litter along the way, you'll get quite a workout, and a half hour of this activity will leave you sweating and breathing hard.

To move up another level, add some jogging or running, however much feels right to you. You can do this either during the entire workout, or only during parts of your excursion. You will find this type of workout quite demanding, much more demanding than just jogging or running.

Obviously, you can approach any workout with a concentration either on basic exercise, endurance, or intensity, or some combination of these. One of my favorite types of workouts starts with gentle walking walking, then advances to power walking, then adds some jogging, then a few wind sprints, then a bit more jogging, and ends with gentle walking again for the cool down phase.

You can add more variety as well as intensity by including bodyweight exercises or calisthenics along the way. For instance, you could do ten jumping jacks each time you find a piece of litter, or add pushups, burpees (a kind of high-intensity cardio exercise consisting of a squat-thrust, pushup, and jump), lunges, or any other exercise you want to do.

The most extreme level of the Litter Patrol Workout would mean running, picking up litter, and doing high-intensity exercises along the way. That's Iron Man level Litter Patrol, and only those in extraordinary shape already should even try this. I tried it only once. It was incredibly difficult and demanding, and I think I'll leave it to the real Litter Patrol Iron Men, if there actually are any. If you aspire to be the first Iron Man of Litter Patrol, and become famous for doing so, you have my full respect and admiration.

12. Litter patrol by bicycle

It may not have occurred to you, but litter patrol by bicycle can be a very effective workout, and can allow you to clean a very large area in little time. Some places have a lot of litter, but the litter is spaced out rather widely. For instance, there is a trail in my neighborhood which always has litter on it, but only about one piece every hundred yards or so. Walking such a route, you would have to walk quite far to pick up much litter. By bicycle, it's a different matter entirely. It's easy to cover ten miles or more by bicycle, stopping occasionally to pick up litter.

It helps to have baskets on the back, or a basket on the handlebars, and a bungee cord or two for keeping bags strapped down. Another advantage of doing litter patrol by bicycle is that riding to a trash can that's a mile away is easier than walking to it. Sometimes I've spent an entire afternoon just riding around picking up litter, filling up my baskets, unloading them at trash cans, and then picking up more litter, etc. It's actually a very interesting way to spend an afternoon, because you end up riding in all kinds of new areas, hunting down the wild and frisky litter.

13. Routes & schedules

If you begin to go out on Litter Patrol, you will soon realize the need to make decisions about routes and schedules. If you patrol an area or a set of areas regularly, you will also get a feel for how frequently those areas need to be patrolled, based on the rate of deposition of new litter. In addition, you will come to instantly recognize the difference between new litter and old litter. New litter is often easier to clean up, but cleaning up old litter generally means that you are making a more substantial, lasting difference. A location with nothing but new litter means it is getting new litter deposited all the time, but when you encounter a site with mostly old litter in it, that means if you clean it up, it will have less litter for longer after you clean it up.

Once you clean up a route or a site, check back some time to see how it's doing. That will give you an idea of how frequently you may want to visit it again. If you clean up a few sites in your area, you will gradually develop a matrix of when to revisit which routes and sites. All of this is of course related to just how clean you want to keep them. I've cleaned up areas with nothing but old litter, knowing that they'd stay pretty clean for another decade or more. I've also lived in areas in which it was clear I should do litter patrol along a heavily used path every week, or even more than once a week.

Near my house there is a large suburban park, a walking trail, and two streets with heavy traffic. I walk around the park once a week, but taking a somewhat different route through the park each time, about an hour each route. The walking trail I patrol a couple of times a week, which only takes about twenty minutes each time. The two streets with heavy traffic I tackle about once a month, which also takes about twenty minutes each time. So every week I'm doing about an hour and three quarters of Litter Patrol exercise, getting other exercise as well, and keeping the neighborhood cleaner than it has ever been.

14. Clothing

What you wear depends in part on your goals, both for the workout and for sites or routes you plan to clean up, but comfortable clothing which allows freedom of movement is essential for the Litter Patrol Workout in any form. You will almost certainly sweat during the workout, and may have to reach in somewhat awkward positions at times. Therefore sweat clothes are close to ideal for most forms of the workout, except during hot weather. If you plan to just stroll along at an easy pace and just pick up litter along the route, the clothes you regularly wear for walks will probably do just fine.

If you will be cleaning up a particularly demanding site, and want to go after all the litter there no matter what, you may need clothing that's a bit more tough, clothing that will be able to withstand brambles and prickers and unexpected abrasion. The heavier clothing means getting hotter inside that clothing, so it's best to schedule such activity on cool days or in the cool of the morning.

You may have the goal of getting some sun during your workout, but doing so in part determines how aggressive and thorough your litter patrol can be. On certain beautiful, sunny days, I head out on litter patrol in just a pair of small shorts in order to get lots of sun, but in that case I limit my litter patrol to just picking things up I find along my route, and certainly not scrambling into the brambles.

15. Gloves

Most people who pick up litter on a regular basis will want to wear gloves of some kind, mainly so that you can feel free to pick up any type of item without getting your hands dirty. There are several options as to gloves, with advantages and disadvantages for each option.

Plastic bag as a glove

The simplest option of all, which also costs nothing, is to use a plastic bag as a glove. You probably already have too many small plastic bags at home, so this is a way of putting them to good use. A bread bag is about the ideal size, because it will also cover your wrist and about half your forearm, so that you can reach into bushes and such with some protection. Plastic bags have several advantages:

- Thin, so you can feel exactly how you are grasping items.
- Transparent, so you can also see the exact position of your fingers, as well as the item you want to pick up.
- Light and compact, so you can easily keep extras in your car trunk or elsewhere.
- Often encountered in exactly the areas which should be cleaned up.

That last point is important, because you may find areas you'd like to clean up, but you don't have any gloves handy. In these cases it's usually easy to find a clean plastic bag that has been discarded in the area itself, and then use that as a glove. Additional plastic bags you find can then be used for holding litter as you collect it.

Rubber gloves

Relatively thin rubber gloves such as dishwashing gloves, gardening gloves or gloves for electrical work are a reasonable option. Rubber gloves are easy to wash, and a high quality pair of rubber gloves will last a long time, even with demanding use. Make sure you get gloves that are big enough to remove easily. It's frustrating to struggle to remove a pair of tight rubber gloves, particularly if the gloves have become at all slippery.

If you can't try the gloves on before you buy them, I would suggest getting a size larger than you think you'll need, just to make sure you can remove them easily. Dishwashing gloves work fairly well, but they tend to be thin and a bit too delicate, tearing too easily. There's not much point in having a glove on with a big tear in it. If you want to use rubber gloves, I would suggest gloves that are thick enough that they won't tear easily. I use a pair of relatively thick rubber gloves designed for electrical work. The have already lasted for years, and are still in great shape. They have a textured surface along the bottom of the fingers, making it easy to grip objects even when the gloves are wet. Needless to say, rubber gloves are much better for reaching into water than leather gloves.

Disposable plastic gloves

Thin, disposable plastic gloves are inexpensive and convenient. They are often available in sets of a dozen or so. Because they are thin, you can feel exactly what your hands are doing. They can be a bit difficult to remove, but since they will be thrown away immediately, you can just tear them off without concern for not tearing them. The drawback to these gloves is that in effect you are creating waste by using them, when the whole idea is to remove and reduce waste. The only time I use disposable plastic gloves is when I invite people to "litter pickup parties," and I want to make sure that everyone will have a pair of gloves to use. Otherwise, I stay away from them because they are wasteful.

Leather gloves

Leather work gloves are also a fine option. One advantage of leather gloves is that they allow moisture to escape, so your hands don't become as sweaty as they do when you use either a plastic bag or rubber gloves. One disadvantage of leather gloves is that it's a bit more difficult to feel exactly how you are making contact with items, but you quickly get used to this. I keep a pair of relatively light leather work gloves handy which are comfortable for me, and easy to remove. If they get dirty, I just wipe them with a rag, because washing with soap or detergent harms the leather. I've used this same pair of leather work gloves for years, and am very happy with them.

One glove, or two?

In many cases I will use only one glove, for the one hand that is making direct contact with the litter. The other hand is then free for other tasks, with full sensation and finer control, and also not getting hot or sweaty inside a glove. It's up to you, but keep in mind that you don't necessarily need to have a glove on each hand, and if wearing only one glove works better for you, then that's what you should do. Michael Jackson will not be offended. He's been dead for some time now.

16. Bags & bag size

It's nice to be ambitious about how much litter you're going to pick up, but there are practical matters to consider regarding the size of the bags you use. I once went on litter patrol with someone who insisted on using a large lawn bag, normally used for collecting piles of leaves. As the bag filled up, he had to drag it around as it got heavier, more bulky and more awkward. This meant he was dragging it across the ground, with a bunch of bulky stuff in it. Eventually the big bag tore open or course, spilling all the litter out, defeating the entire point of his litter patrol. So size does matter after all, at least where litter bag size is concerned.

In most situations, it's best to use fairly small bags, even if you end up using several of them. Most items of litter are small, and also can be crushed before placing in the bag. If you get used to compacting items with either your feet or your hands before placing them in the bag, you can fit a lot of litter in a fairly small bag. Small bags are also easier to carry because they are lighter, and less bulky. In general, I only use the extra plastic bags that build up from shopping, that is bread bags, produce bags, clothing bags, and random other small bags.

One technique which works well for small bags if you fill up a lot of them during a major patrol is to just leave them in obvious places along your route when they fill up, then go pick them all up as a last step, possibly tossing all the small bags into one larger bag if necessary. This is much easier than trying to hold onto multiple full small bags while you're on patrol, which frankly is close to impossible, as well as mighty annoying.

Certain sites are already stocked with bags you can use. The thin white grocery bags with handles are everywhere as of this writing, unfortunately. Those bags will do fine for litter patrol, although they tend to be rather too open at the top, such that items can spill out if you're not careful. One technique I use is to stuff smaller items of litter inside somewhat larger items–gum wrappers, cigarette butts, plastic cutlery inside larger paper coffee cups, for instance. This way all the small items are better contained, so there are fewer total items that can spill out accidentally.

I would strongly encourage you to make use of the extra plastic bags around your house for litter patrol, rather than buying bags just for the purpose. Most of us end up throwing out large numbers of plastic bags of various sizes during the year, in fact more than even the most dedicated litter patrollers could use. Many of those bags are perfect for litter patrol, and actually better than the thin garbage bags, which tear easily. Save some money, save some resources, and head out on patrol!

17. Small backpack

A small backpack or daypack can make collecting litter much easier, particularly in areas where there are no trash cans, or trash cans are few and far between. When you've filled up one of the bags and a trash can is not nearby, just stuff the full bag into the pack. Most day packs can fit several small bags full of litter, particularly if you make a point of compressing each piece of litter before placing it in the bag. If you are at all concerned about keeping the inside of your bag completely away from contact even with the plastic bag full of litter, it's a simple matter to line the pack with a medium sized plastic bag, so that none of the litter bags actually touch the inside of the pack. Wearing a pack is also handy because you can keep a bunch of small plastic bags either lashed to the pack or in an open side pocket, such that even while wearing the pack you should be able to reach back and grab another plastic bag. Another tip is to bring a set of small metal ties with you, so that you can seal the top of each bag when you place it in the pack, so that litter doesn't spill out inside the pack.

17. Grabber, or no grabber?

A "grabber" is a device which extends your reach by a couple of feet or more. It is a short pole, with a squeeze handle on one end, and a simple pair of "fingers" on the other, usually fitted with small rubber cups for a better grip. Squeeze the handle, and the fingers come together at the other end. Using a grabber, you can pick items up without bending down, and also reach items you otherwise would not be able to reach, such as items in bushes, or crevices, or in the water. A grabber can be handy, particularly for anyone who has trouble bending over. It can also be a bit frustrating however, because even the best grabber can't grip certain things very well, and is nowhere near as versatile or as sensitive or as strong as your hand. Trying to pick up a glass bottle covered with slime out of the water can be frustrating, for instance.

I generally only use a grabber for sites I know contain items that would be difficult to reach without one. A grabber is great for sites with litter stuck far back in bushes or up in trees, as well as sites in which there are many items in the water fairly close by. When using a grabber, sometimes it's easy to stuff an item into a bag directly with the end of the grabber, but other times it's necessary to remove the item from the end of the grabber with the other hand. This means that it can make sense to wear only one glove, on the hand that is not holding the grabber.

If you're thinking of buying a grabber, keep in mind that it's handy having a grabber around at home for other reasons, like retrieving socks that have fallen behind the dryer, frisbees stuck in trees, and so on. If you do buy a grabber, get a very good one. The cheap grabbers are terrible, and will break so soon they're not worth buying. I bought a cheap grabber initially, thinking I was saving money. It was so flimsy it broke after less than an hour. I then shopped carefully for a high quality grabber, which has served me well for many years now.

18. Hygiene

Most litter is completely innocuous. It's been baking in the disinfectant of the sun for weeks, and may be a little bit dirty, but then so are gardening tools. Still, some litter is pretty icky, and the worst of such litter should definitely be left alone.

It's completely up to you what you pick up and what you don't, and whether you wear gloves, or just use your hands. Some times I wear gloves, other times not. It depends what the site is like, and what kind of litter I expect to encounter. If it's a yucky site, I'll definitely wear gloves. If the site contains mostly aluminum cans, food wrappers and paper coffee cups, I'll just use my hands.

If you reach into bushes or brambles, keep in mind that if you're not careful, you can get scratched on your arms or face. If you are wearing shorts, you can also get scratched on your legs. Wading into dirty water without protection for your skin is a bad idea. I have cleaned up some sites that required me to wade into the water a bit, but I always did so wearing strong synthetic pants and socks, with boots on. If you do get scratched, wash the scratch and apply disinfectant as soon as possible.

19. Trash cans & routes

As you gain experience with the Litter Patrol Workout, as well as with specific sites, you will begin to see opportunities for simplifying and making easier aspects of your routine. For instance, if there are trash cans along your route, you will definitely want to discard what you have collected into the closest trash can, in order not to be burdened as you proceed further. One approach to this is to bring a good number of small bags, then deposit the entire bag and its contents into a trash can, and start with a another empty bag. A different approach is to bring only one or two bags, and then discard only the contents of the bag into the trash can, and then use the same bag again. I've gone out on long, elaborate patrols in areas with trash cans close by, using only one bag, which I just empty completely every time I am near a trash can.

Depending on the availability and proximity of trash cans, you may choose to fill up a small bag, leave it along the route, and fill up additional bags and leave them along the route as well, and then make one sweep back to pick up all the bags at once, and put them in the trash. I have done this when backpacking, for instance. When I head in to a site, my pack is full, so I fill up small bags with litter and leave them in obvious places along the trail. On the way out from the site, my pack is lighter because I've eaten all the food in it, so it's easy to pick up the bags and either stuff them in the pack or lash them to the pack. I also once participated in a roadside cleanup, and our procedure was to fill up rather large bags while walking, leave them by the side of the road, then at the end drive by and pick them all up in one swoop. But the same procedure can be applied to cleaning up an urban or suburban park, or a large roadside pullout. It's easy to just grab all the bags at the very end, but it's not at all easy to try to hold on to multiple bags as you pick up litter.

Choosing a site which already contains trash cans can make the entire process simpler and more convenient, but as you gain experience you'll find yourself naturally strategizing ahead of time, no matter what the site, about how you will most efficiently collect, consolidate and dispose of the litter.

20. Types of sites

Since litter is nearly ubiquitous, there are many different types of sites in which you can get a workout. Some of them are obvious, but some may not have occurred to you. I have experience with so many different types of sites that I'd like to offer guidance on some of them.

Suburban streets

Suburban streets can make for a good workout, especially if you include some power walking and a bit of jogging. Items of litter tend to be widely spaced, and there usually are not many trash cans along the route. This can mean that you end up carrying small bags of litter over fairly long distances before being able to dispose of them. However, if there is roadside trash pickup on a particular day, you can choose a route and time such that you can toss your bags of litter into the bins set out by the road. You may also know of dumpsters nearby, perhaps behind restaurants or grocery stores, where you can stash the trash. It's a good idea to ask permission from the establishment first of course. Once you tell them that you're cleaning up trash in the area almost everyone will happily agree, because they like their neighborhood to be clean too. If it isn't easy to find the owner of the dumpster, it's generally fine to just toss in your bags of trash. If someone questions you, you're ready with a very good answer.

Keep in mind that you don't need to confine your activities to your local neighborhood. It's an easy matter to scope out a place to park in an area you're not familiar with, then explore the new area on foot. This is a great way of expanding your knowledge of your region in fine detail.

Suburban streets are an excellent opportunity for litter patrol by bicycle, both because litter is generally sparse on suburban streets, and because on a bicycle it's a simple matter to ride some distance to a new section of town, and start your patrol from there.

City parks

Most city parks are a slam dunk for litter patrol, and I mean that literally, because they have trash cans on site. If the trash cans are open at the top, you can make a game of trying to lob pieces of litter in from a distance, getting extra exercise and practicing your coordination and accuracy. In many city parks you don't even have to bring a plastic bag because the trash cans are so close.

Most city parks are also excellent sites for adding other exercises to your routine. For instance, if there are benches, you can do angled pushups against a bench. Angled pushups are easier than regular pushups, and you don't have to get down on the ground to do them. You can also do "step ups" onto the bench, alternating legs. Study the site for opportunities to add exercises you know, or invent new exercises based on what you find at the site. Some city parks even include exercise equipment, so you can get a double workout, if you so choose.

Suburban parks

Some suburban parks are very pleasant and even beautiful, and make a wonderful environment for the Litter Patrol Workout. Those parks which get heavy use on the weekends generally have plenty of litter on Monday morning. In some of these parks the trash cans may be a bit widely spaced, so it's a good idea to scope out the location of the cans, so that you can plan an efficient and convenient route accordingly.

Parking lots

Nearly every parking lot has some trash in it. Parking lots are generally not the most pleasant sites for a Litter Patrol Workout, but it's still helpful to clean up a parking lot for the sake of others. Most parking lots have trash cans near the entrance to stores or businesses. If you are traveling by car, keep in mind that every parking lot is an opportunity to get out of the car and get some exercise. I get very antsy if I have to sit in a car for more than a couple of hours, and just getting up and stretching my legs is not enough relief for me. Therefore I have cleaned up many a parking lot on my travels, and have been thankful for the opportunity to exercise between bouts of sitting on my butt in the car.

Rest stops

Rest stops represent one of the best opportunities for litter patrol, and for exercise while traveling. Many rest stops have quite a lot of litter, particularly at the edges. They also always have trash cans, making litter patrol convenient. My usual routine at a rest stop if I am traveling is to spend about 15-20 minutes cleaning the site up, just enough to get my blood moving and my muscles stretched out, so that going a few more hours in the car is more comfortable.

Roadside pullouts

Thoroughly cleaning up an otherwise beautiful roadside pullout that has been trashed is one of the nicest things you can do for your fellow travelers, as well as one of the most satisfying types of Litter Patrol Workouts. It's hard not to be appalled when you stop in a roadside pullout under a beautiful grove of trees by a gorgeous little stream and find piles of beer cans, fast food containers, whiskey bottles and plastic bags everywhere. What the hell were these people thinking, trashing a beautiful place like this? The best thing to do, the most noble thing to do, the only way of solving the problem, is to pitch right in and clean the whole damn place up yourself. When you're done, you will be absolutely amazed how much better it looks.

Sometimes a roadside pullout will have so much trash that you do need somewhat larger plastic bags to deal with it all. I always bring a few medium size garbage bags with me when I travel, just in case I encounter this kind of situation. I also make sure there is some space left in the car for a few full bags, usually in the trunk.

Depending on the size and condition of the site, it may take a while to get it completely clean. If you can make the time, bringing a beautiful natural site back to a pristine condition is deeply satisfying, and almost miraculous. You will have to decide how much you are willing to do. When I encounter a truly special site that has been hurt by people, I simply have to put it right. If that takes an hour or two, or even more, that's fine with me. When I do this, I am full of love. I fall in love with the site, and enjoy every moment, every detail. It's as though I am healing someone, someone I love very much, and every piece of ugly trash I pick up is helping my friend return to good health, and good spirits. At the end I usually spend some additional time just enjoying how much better the site looks, before driving on.

Trails

There are many kinds of trails, but nearly all of them have some litter on them, whether widely or closely spaced. Some people object to the idea of picking up litter when they are out "enjoying nature." They feel that dealing with litter ruins their experience. I have a big problem with that attitude, for a few reasons. First, it's completely selfish. It means that you're so concerned with your own experience that you can't stop a few times, pick up a bit of litter, and make the next person's experience a bit better. Second, it offers no solution whatsoever. Many trails are not regularly cleaned up, so any litter is going to remain an eyesore indefinitely, unless someone traveling the trail picks it up. Third, it calls into question your relationship with nature. You love nature so much that you're not willing to take a simple action to protect and preserve it? That's a one-way kind of love that isn't real love at all. Real love means being willing to make an effort to make things right.

It's a simple matter to bring a couple of small plastic bags with you when you head out on the trail. Just stuff one in your pocket, and another in any pack or bag you may be carrying. When you encounter some litter, get the bag out of your pocket and start filling up the bag. Depending on whether the litter is widely or closely spaced in general, I will either just hold the bag, or keep it in my pack, or lash it to my pack for easy access. If you will be coming out along the same trail and have filled up two bags or more, you can use the trick I mentioned earlier of just leaving the bags along the trail in obvious spots, and picking them up on your way out.

Beaches

While beaches may be inspiring and beautiful, they are not always the best place for the Litter Patrol Workout. It depends on the qualities of the beach, and the type of litter found there. In sand that gives way under your feet, walking itself can be very tiring, especially for your ankles. Harder sand near the water's edge can be easier to walk on, but is not necessarily where most of the litter is found. Some of the nicest beaches are also remote, which means that there are very few trash cans. In addition, some of the "litter" found on beaches may consist of large, bulky items which you definitely cannot haul away easily yourself, and may be both wet, slippery, and quite gross. I tend to confine my litter patrol to beaches with trash cans nearby, and I leave the bulkier items for official beach cleanups, in which a crew can easily handle and haul away just about anything.

Vacant Lots

Many vacant lots would be quite attractive, if not for the litter all over them. Cleaning up a vacant lot can be a very satisfying experience, particularly if you're willing to thoroughly clean up the entire lot. Taking before and after pictures makes the experience even better, and provides an impressive way to share what you've accomplished. However, it's easy to underestimate the time it will take to clean up a vacant lot. What looks like only a half hour's work can stretch into two hours or more.

Another issue with vacant lots which comes up frequently is access. Many of these lots have cyclone fencing around them, making it challenging even to get into the lot itself. I've cleaned up quite a few vacant lots, but only lots which I can enter easily. If you find a large lot you'd like to clean up but the lot is fenced off, the best choices are either to choose another site or, if you're truly serious, find and contact the owner and put together a small crew to clean it up. Completely cleaning up a lot and making it look great, and then sitting down with a good sandwich and cold beverage is a truly satisfying experience, especially among friends or other dedicated litter picker uppers.

Roads

Some roads are terribly trashed. Roadside cleanup is a noble effort, but actually doesn't make for the best workout, and there can be an issue of safety, depending on the nature of the road. If you do want to clean up a section of road, I would suggest putting together a small crew, wearing dayglow jackets or vests, and parking a car on the shoulder behind where you will be working, in order to alert other drivers, and form a barrier between you and oncoming traffic. The usual procedure in this case is to use medium size plastic bags, and leave them on the far side of the shoulder of the road when they're full. As a final step, drive by and pick up all the bags in one sweep. This is much easier than walking the bags one by one back to the car, and then walking back again to pick up more litter.

Highways

I strongly recommend against going on litter patrol on highways of any kind, even those with only light traffic. It's generally not safe, and definitely is not safe if you are working alone. The only time this activity is safe is when a large crew is working, with a large "follow truck" behind them, forming a barrier between the crew and traffic. It's too bad highways are not safe for this kind of activity, because highways are some of the most heavily littered environments, but it's best to leave cleanup of highways to the work crews in the bright orange suits, with the bright orange plastic cones, and the big orange truck to protect them.

Railroad tracks

Walking by the railroad tracks can be a very interesting experience. In every case you will see an area from a perspective you have probably never seen it before, and you will discover things you never even knew existed in your locale. I've done this many times, both on litter patrol and just exploring. Contrary to popular belief, as long as you listen for trains, walking by the tracks is quite safe. It's easy to hear a train more than half a mile away, so you have a long time to just step well away from the tracks, and then wave to the driver as the train rumbles past.

If you do choose to do litter patrol by the tracks, you are likely to find some of the most unusual items. It's wildly unpredictable, and sometimes you will find the most amazing, weird and wonderful things. One issue at these sites is that some of the items are rather large, so you have to make decisions about which of them you are going to not deal with at all. For these sites, it's actually better to bring a set of larger, tougher plastic bags, due to the nature of some of what you may find. My procedure is to fill up the bags one by one, leave them well off to the side of the tracks one by one, then when I've gone as far as I want to, begin walking back and picking them up two by two, one in each hand for balance. That last part can give you quite the upper body workout in itself. Do this enough, and you will have shoulders of steel, as hard as the railroad tracks.

It's easy to fill up a bunch of bags when walking by the tracks, more bags than you want to deal with disposing of yourself. In this case it's a good idea to scope out the nearest train station and its trash cans, and have a small sign prepared with an explanation that the litter is from the tracks. Leave that sign pinned to the bags of trash, next to the regular trash cans, so that station management will know it's not from someone dumping their own personal trash.

21. Adopt a site, freelance, or both

It can be nice to adopt a particular site, visit it regularly, enjoy getting to know the site in intimate detail over multiple visits, and take pride in keeping it clean. You can also "freelance," taking on whatever sites you encounter that appeal to you. Both approaches have their charms. I like to do both. In my neighborhood, I go out on litter patrol regularly over about four square blocks, but I am also on the lookout for other sites locally, and I do litter patrol while traveling as well.

22. Types of litter & how to deal with them

As you gain experience on litter patrol, you will encounter many different types of items, and will begin to wonder what is the best way to deal with some of them. In the next section I'll give my recommendations on how to deal with the most commonly encountered items. You are free to make your own choices, of course. If you think of a way of dealing with any of the types of litter listed below that is better than what I recommend, by all means do it your way.

Aluminum cans

An aluminum can is mostly empty space, and is very light. One good stomp with your foot will completely flatten an aluminum can down to a tenth its original size, or less. This makes it very easy to carry a lot of aluminum cans, and also to place them in a separate bag for recycling, if you're so inclined. It's a good idea to bring a rag so that you can wipe off any dirty can before giving it the stomp treatment. Some cans may also have dirt or debris inside. A good technique for rinsing such cans is to wait until you find a bottle or can with some fluid in it, and use that fluid to give the dirty can a rinse. I often find half-full water bottles, and use the water from these bottles to rinse off other items.

Glass bottles

Obviously, glass bottles can be put in the recycling bin, and more and more often you will find recycling bins in such locations as city and suburban parks. As with aluminum cans, a rag and a bit of fluid from other containers can get these items reasonably clean in a snap. If you can't find a recycling bin close by, but there are trash cans, it's not a bad idea to leave the glass bottles at the base of the trash can instead of tossing them in. Some municipalities will keep the recyclable items separate during collection, if you make it easy for them, and if you are in an area in which there is a deposit on glass bottles, recycling scavengers will snap the bottles up in no time.

Plastic bags

You will definitely find plastic bags of various kinds in your patrols. Some of these bags can be used for gathering litter. In fact, even if you start your patrol without a plastic bag, chances are you will soon find one. The most common plastic bags are the whites ones from supermarkets, medium size, with handles. You will also find many other kinds, of various size and thickness. Though your first inclination may be to stuff these bags in with all the other litter, it's often a good idea to collect them and keep them either in your pockets, or in a small pack if you are wearing one. Extra bags can come in handy during a patrol in case you find more litter than you were expecting, or want to extend your patrol. Another reason to keep extra bags separate is that you may want to either bring them home to have extras, or may want to put them in the recycling bin.

Plastic breaking up in the sun

Occasionally you will find pieces of plastic of various thickness which have been out in the sun a long time, and are beginning to break up into smaller pieces. Some of these items will begin to completely fall apart as you try to pick them up. Each additional piece you try to pick up may then break up into even smaller pieces. This can be quite frustrating. In some cases you can pick up the major pieces by using a much lighter touch so that they don't break up when you grasp them. In other cases it's better to get out the bag you're using to collect the litter, and use a sweeping motion to get all of the pieces to go into the bag at once, even as they break up further from the impact of the sweeping motion. If the plastic is thin and is breaking easily into tiny pieces, really the best thing to do is to just brush it vigorously with your hand so that it breaks up completely, and is blown away by the wind. There's nothing wrong with doing this, because there was no way to pick up the plastic anyway, so it was going to stay in the environment no matter what you did. Might as well disperse it into tiny pieces and let the elements break it down completely.

Plastic cups

In order to save space, plastic cups can be stacked together before being placed in the bag you are using to gather litter. Unlike aluminum cans and paper cups, plastic cups do not compact well at all, instead springing back partially, into awkward shapes. What I do is put small items inside the first cup I find, then stack any additional cups I find onto the bottom of the first cup. This way I keep total size to a minimum, while also confining smaller items so that they don't fall out and have to be collected again. Most plastic cups can be put in the recycling bin, so if you do intend to put recyclables in the closest bin, stacking the plastic cups makes it easier to keep them all together.

Paper cups

Paper cups can either be compacted with a good whomp of your foot, or stacked together if you find a lot of them of similar sizes. They can also be used to keep the smaller items confined, just as with plastic cups, and as with plastic cups they can be put in the recycling bin if that's part of your patrol.

Styrofoam cups

These cups are prevalent, a bit difficult to deal with, and in general should not be put in the recycling bin. Technically styrofoam can be recycled, and you may find the "recyclable" logo and a recycling type number on the bottom, but most styrofoam cups you will find have been contaminated with food waste, and would be rejected by a recycling center for that reason. It's best to just collect these, stuff them in the bag, and throw them out.

Organic matter

I've found it's best to deal with most organic matter by allowing it to decompose on the site, but inconspicuously. Things like apple cores, orange and banana peels, even watermelon rinds, I either throw way back in the bushes where they'll never be seen, or I kick a little hole in the ground with the end of my shoe and cover the item with a bit of dirt or leaves. Most organic matter will decompose rapidly, particularly if kept wet, so all you are doing is helping it along, well out of sight. I think this is better than filling your bag with partly nonorganic items, partly organic items, the mixing together of which just makes the nonorganic items which you may want to put in the recycling bin dirtier. Let the organic stuff rot on site, but out of sight, I say.

Clothing

In your patrols, you will eventually find clothing of various kinds, in various conditions. If you do find clothing and it is in good shape, you have a couple of options. The most noble option is to bring it home, wash it, and donate it to a thrift store. That's what I do. I've found a whole lot of clothing, and in most cases if it's in reasonable shape I'll either just sling it over my shoulder, or put it in the pack, if I'm wearing one. I feel very good about saving all those clothes from the landfill, and helping to provide clothing for the needy. Another option is to leave the clothing in an obvious place, such as directly next to a trash bin, in the hope that someone else will either want it, or will pick it up and bring it home, either to wear, or to donate. The third option is to just throw the clothing away, though it's really a shame to do that, if the clothing could be used by someone else. As with every other aspect of the Litter Patrol Workout, the choice is up to you.

Stuff you probably don't want to deal with

You will definitely find stuff you won't want to deal with. My advice is to not deal with it. You're already doing good in the world. No need to be a martyr about it. Just move on and continue picking up the stuff you don't mind picking up, and feel good about doing so.

23. Separation of litter types, or not

If you begin to go out on litter patrol regularly, you will soon encounter a quandary; you are doing something very good by picking up litter, but keeping recyclables separate from trash makes the entire process unwieldy and a bit of a burden. Even just trying to carry two bags instead of one, with one of the bags for recyclables, can feel like an awkward juggling act. It's a perfectly valid option to decide that you're going to do good by picking up litter, but you're not going to extend your efforts to separating the recyclables. That's a perfectly acceptable choice, since you're already doing so much good. Another option is to quickly pick out the recyclables when you get to a trash can, and leave them conspicuously at the base of the trash can. In communities where there are deposits on aluminum cans and glass bottles, those items will be snapped up quickly. A third option, if you do want to make sure the recyclables get into a recycling bin, is to wear a small pack, and stuff the recyclables in a second bag inside the pack. This does mean stopping occasionally to open the pack, but you can reduce the number of times you have to do this by tucking a few items under your arm or in a small bag for a while, and only stopping to put them in the pack when you've gathered a few of them.

One situation which makes separating recyclables easy is if you stop at a roadside pullout. In most roadside pullouts you will find lots of aluminum cans and glass bottles. Since the location is relatively small, and you have your car right there, it's an easy matter to separate the recyclables with minimal extra walking. Then just keep the recyclables in your trunk until you either get home, or happen upon a recycling bin.

24. Setting limits

It's important to define clearly in your patrols what you are and aren't going to do. As mentioned above, you are under no obligation to pick up all kinds of materials, under no obligation to keep recyclables separate, and under no obligation to do the work in any particular way, or with any particular thoroughness. If you decide you're only going to pick up the easy, obvious stuff, that's perfectly fine, and I thank you for doing so. If you decide you're only going to spend fifteen minutes, or even just five minutes, that's five minutes or fifteen minutes of doing good that most people will never choose to do, and again I thank you for your work. Whatever you choose to do, just be clear with yourself about the limits you choose to set, and proud that you're being helpful at all.

25. Treasure

If you go out on litter patrol regularly, you will eventually find "treasure." I have found all kinds of wonderful, crazy stuff. One item was a large, high-quality hard plastic model of a lighthouse, complete with battery-powered foghorn. It was designed as a cookie jar, such that any time someone flipped the top open and reached in for a cookie, the foghorn would sound, letting everyone in the house know that someone was having a cookie. I took it home, gave it a thorough cleaning, put some fresh batteries in it, and made a short video of the foghorn going off, which I posted on YouTube before donating this weird, charming device to a thrift store. I've also found baseballs in perfect shape, tennis racquets, a large pure wool overcoat in perfect condition (original cost at least $150), perfectly good shoes, notepads and pens, and much more. I'm a dedicated minimalist and already own everything I want, so I always just clean the "treasure" up and either donate it to a thrift store or leave it out somewhere conspicuous with a note inviting people to take it home. But if you find something abandoned while you're out on litter patrol and you want to take it home yourself, it's yours, and you're welcome to it.

26. Keep bags and gloves in your trunk

I like to be ready to clean up a site when I'm traveling by car, so I keep a pair of gloves and about a dozen medium size plastic bags in the trunk. This means that whenever I see a site that could use a cleanup, I can stop without hesitation, knowing I've got the basic tools of the trade. It's a good idea to either get bags with a "cinch strip" at the top to keep the bags closed when they're full, or to bring along some bag ties. Either way, it's important to tie the bags closed so that nothing gets loose.

I mentioned this before, but one of my favorite types of litter patrol site is scenic roadside pullouts. I absolutely love making a beautiful site that has been trashed pristine again, and I am willing to work hard to do so. In the process I get a good workout, which is far superior to just getting out of the car for a few minutes on a long drive.

27. Wash up afterward, friend

Even if you wear gloves, you're going to get a little dirty, or at least a little sweaty when you go out on patrol. Make it a point to wash up immediately afterward. I usually schedule patrols so that I take a shower as soon as I get back. If you do get really dirty, be proud. You earned that dirt.

28. Don't worry, be happy

As you deal with litter on your patrols, you may begin to feel a certain level of outrage at the litterbugs of the world. You may begin to be seriously puzzled as to how people can be such slobs. You may even begin to get very angry at all the inconsiderate creeps who just toss their garbage everywhere. Every piece of litter may just increase your anger, and your outrage.

Don't go down that path. It's not worth it, and there's nothing you can do about it. As I mentioned at the very beginning of this little book, the litterbugs are a relatively small, probably completely incorrigible proportion of the population. You can't change them, so don't let them change you. Just enjoy the work, take pride in doing it, get a good workout, and be on your merry way. I dedicated this book to all the litterbug who have kept me in such good shape all my life, and I meant it. If only a tiny fraction of the population went out on litter patrol regularly, there would be no litter anywhere, and those people would be in better shape. Just be one of those people, and be happy about it.

29. Enjoy the scenery

Wherever you go on litter patrol, always remember to enjoy the scenery. Don't get so fixated on the ground and on picking up litter that you forget to look up and admire and enjoy everything else. If you want to specialize in cleaning up beautiful natural locations that have been abused, you will have some truly wonderful scenery to enjoy.

One of the best ways of arranging and scheduling litter patrol is to choose a location you like, estimate the time it will take to clean it up, and bring a picnic lunch with you. This way you will be able to enjoy your lunch while also enjoying the newly pristine, beautiful scenery. There is little better in this life than a good sandwich, a cold beverage, a clean napkin, a sweaty body from a great workout, and a setting which you just restored to its natural beauty.

30. Greetings, thanks & honks

Believe me, if you go out on litter patrol, you will be noticed. Many people will just look at you in wonder. Others will give you a big greeting, and big thanks. If you are cleaning up a roadside, you can expect some honks and waves. All of this is very nice, and I'd encourage you to be openly friendly about all of it. I love when people honk and wave. It's totally fun, and sometimes I just wave a piece of litter at them, grinning like the do-gooding fool that I am.

31. Take pride in your work

Remember, you are doing a great service for everyone who encounters any site you clean up. You are making the world a little bit better, in part by spreading a good example. Take pride in your work. Do a great job of it. Work to become better at it, and take pride in that, too. Don't brag, but don't be shy about letting others know what you are doing. This hobby is much more useful than a whole lot of other hobbies I can think of.

32. Take the time to admire your work

I'd encourage you, at the end of your patrols, to take a few minutes to admire your work. This can be an important emotional payoff that makes you feel great, and makes you look forward to further cleanup projects. If you cleaned up a stretch of street, take a final stroll down the section you cleaned up, and enjoy how much better it looks. If you cleaned up a natural area that was trashed, sit down and just admire the area for a few moments, and think about how much you helped. If you cleaned up a little park, take a few minutes to wander around and take in all the details that look so much better, thanks to the work you did. This is important. Treat yourself to this experience every time you can.

33. Take before and after pictures & share them

For certain sites, particularly beautiful sites that have been trashed, it's a great idea to take before and after pictures, and share them with friends, family and acquaintances. Post them on Facebook, Instagram or other services, and explain what you did. Let people know the exact location, so that they can check out the location and check out your work themselves.   Obviously, another motivation for doing this is to spread a good example, and see whether other people might be interested in either joining you for patrols, or taking up the activity themselves.

34. Organize group outings as social events

I would encourage you to invite other people out on your patrols. You can present this any way you'd like. You can just say "I'm going out on a walk, would you like to come along? I pick up litter along the way, too." Two or three people can clean up small to medium size locations very quickly, and two or three people walking together can completely clean up a trail or roadside or park path easily, while also conversing easily along the way.

As in the previous section, please post pictures of your work, particularly if you have gotten a small group together for cleanups. This can be very inspiring to other people, and make them interested in participating. Spread the word!

35. Thank you!

Finally, thank you so much for reading this little book. I wrote it as a labor of love, because I know that together, we can make the world a little nicer, a little more beautiful, and a lot more inspiring. Thank you, and perhaps see you out on patrol some time!

www.ingramcontent.com/pod-product-compliance
Lightning Source LLC
Chambersburg PA
CBHW060704280326
41933CB00012B/2301